The Beginner's Guide to Psilocybin

A Comprehensive Companion for Safe and Transformative Journeys

David Morales Jr.

To those who seek to explore the depths of their mind
and the world around them, this guide is for you.

Table of Contents

Introduction

Understanding Psilocybin

Psilocybin is a naturally occurring psychedelic compound found in certain mushrooms, often referred to as "magic mushrooms." These mushrooms have a rich history of use in various cultures around the world, particularly in indigenous communities in Central and South America. They have been revered for centuries for their spiritual, medicinal, and therapeutic properties.

When consumed, psilocybin is converted into psilocin in the body, which primarily affects the serotonin receptors in the brain. This interaction leads to significant changes in perception, mood, and cognition. Individuals often report experiencing enhanced sensory perception, vivid visual and auditory hallucinations, and a profound sense of interconnectedness with the world around them.

The altered states of consciousness induced by psilocybin can facilitate deep personal insights, emotional healing, and a new perspective on life. Many people describe their experiences as mystical or transcendental, often leading to lasting positive changes in their outlook and behavior. Research has shown that psilocybin can help alleviate symptoms of depression, anxiety, PTSD, and addiction, making it a promising tool for mental health therapy.

Psilocybin journeys are highly individual, with each person's experience being unique. Factors such as dosage, setting, mindset, and individual psychology all play crucial roles in shaping the experience. While some may encounter challenging moments during their journey, these often lead to significant breakthroughs and personal growth when navigated with the right support and preparation.

As you explore the world of psilocybin, it is essential to approach it with respect, mindfulness, and an open heart. By understanding its effects, preparing adequately, and integrating the insights gained, you can unlock the transformative potential of psilocybin and embark on a journey of self-discovery, healing, and enlightenment.

Benefits of Psilocybin

Research has demonstrated numerous benefits of psilocybin, including:

Mental Health:

One of the most significant areas of research on psilocybin is its potential to alleviate mental health issues. Studies have shown that psilocybin can lead to a substantial reduction in symptoms of depression, anxiety, and PTSD. Unlike traditional treatments, psilocybin can provide long-lasting relief after just a few sessions. This is thought to be due to its ability to foster new perspectives and insights, allowing individuals to process and integrate traumatic experiences more effectively. Additionally, psilocybin has been found to reduce the fear response, making it particularly useful for those with PTSD.

Creativity:

Psilocybin is known to enhance creative thinking and problem-solving skills. People often report experiencing a heightened sense of imagination and the ability to think outside the box. This can be attributed to the way psilocybin disrupts typical patterns of brain activity, allowing for novel connections and ideas to emerge. Artists, writers, and other creative professionals have utilized psilocybin to overcome creative blocks and explore new artistic directions. The compound's ability to enhance sensory perception also contributes to more vivid and inspiring experiences, which can be channeled into creative endeavors.

Well-being:

Psilocybin can significantly increase one's sense of connection, peace, and overall well-being. Many people describe a profound feeling of unity with others and the universe, often referred to as a "mystical experience." These experiences can lead to a deeper appreciation for life, nature, and relationships, fostering a sense of gratitude and contentment. Research has indicated that psilocybin can improve emotional regulation and resilience, helping individuals cope better with life's challenges. This enhanced sense of well-being can persist long after the psilocybin experience, contributing to sustained mental health improvements.

Spiritual Growth:

Psilocybin has been used for centuries in religious and shamanic rituals to deepen spiritual understanding and personal insight. Modern people often report similar experiences of spiritual awakening and enlightenment. Psilocybin can dissolve the ego, allowing individuals to connect with their inner selves and the greater universe on a profound level. This can lead to transformative experiences that reshape one's beliefs, values, and sense of purpose. Many people find that psilocybin helps them explore existential questions and develop a more meaningful and fulfilling spiritual practice.

Additional Benefits:

Neuroplasticity:

Neuroplasticity, the brain's ability to reorganize and form new neural connections. This can enhance learning, memory, and cognitive flexibility, allowing individuals to adapt more readily to new situations and challenges. Neuroplasticity is also associated with recovery from brain injuries and the mitigation of age-related cognitive decline.

Default Mode Network (DMN):

Psilocybin has a profound effect on the brain's default mode network (DMN), a network of interacting brain regions that is active when the mind is at rest and not focused on the outside world. The DMN is associated with self-referential thoughts, rumination, and the sense of self. Overactivity in the DMN is linked to conditions such as depression and anxiety. Psilocybin reduces activity in the DMN, leading to a decrease in rigid, self-focused thinking and enabling a more fluid and interconnected state of consciousness. This alteration can facilitate profound personal insights and a break from negative thought patterns.

Addiction Treatment:

Emerging research suggests that psilocybin may be effective in treating various forms of addiction, including alcoholism, nicotine addiction, and opioid dependence. By disrupting entrenched patterns of behavior and thought, psilocybin can help individuals gain new insights into their addictive behaviors and develop healthier coping mechanisms.

Enhanced Empathy & Interpersonal Relationships:

Psilocybin can enhance empathy and improve interpersonal relationships. People often report a greater ability to understand and connect with others, fostering more compassionate and supportive relationships. This enhanced empathy can lead to improved communication, conflict resolution, and overall relationship satisfaction.

Pain Management:

Some studies have indicated that psilocybin can help manage chronic pain conditions. By altering the perception of pain and reducing emotional distress associated with it, psilocybin can provide relief for those suffering from chronic pain, fibromyalgia, and other debilitating conditions.

Conclusion:

The benefits of psilocybin are wide-ranging and profound, offering potential relief for various mental health conditions, fostering creativity, enhancing well-being, and promoting spiritual growth. By impacting the brain's default mode network, psilocybin can disrupt negative thought patterns and enable transformative personal insights. As research continues to uncover its therapeutic potential, psilocybin stands to become an invaluable tool for personal development and healing. By approaching its use with respect and mindfulness, individuals can harness the transformative power of psilocybin to improve their lives and the lives of those around them.

Legal Considerations

The legal status of psilocybin varies widely across the globe. In some places, it has been decriminalized or legalized for medical use, while in others, it remains illegal. It is crucial to understand and comply with the laws in your area to ensure safe and legal usage.

In the United States, psilocybin is considered a Schedule I controlled substance, making it illegal under federal law. However, cities like Denver and Oakland have decriminalized its use, and Oregon has legalized psilocybin therapy under regulated conditions.

Disclaimer

This guide is intended for informational purposes only. The author does not advocate illegal activities and is not responsible for any individual's use of psilocybin, including their dosing and the outcomes of their experiences. Always consult with a healthcare professional and adhere to local laws and regulations.

Part One: Preparation

Setting Intentions

Importance of Intentions

Defining your intentions before embarking on a psilocybin journey is crucial. Intentions are the purposes or goals you set for the experience. They can range from seeking personal insights, healing, and spiritual growth, to simply exploring consciousness. Setting clear intentions can significantly enhance your psilocybin journey, providing direction and purpose. Intentions act as a compass, guiding you towards meaningful insights and experiences. Clear intentions help guide the experience, providing a focus that can influence the journey's direction and outcomes..

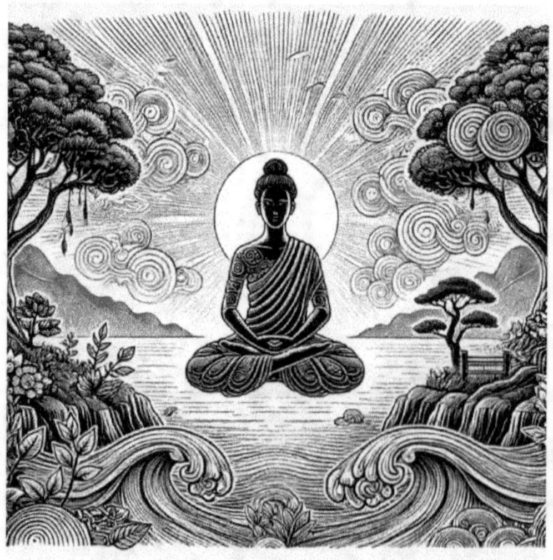

How to Set Intentions

Reflect on what you hope to gain from the experience. Write down your intentions and revisit them before the journey. They can be related to personal growth, healing, creativity, or understanding yourself better.

Examples of Positive Intentions:

1. To gain clarity on a personal issue:

  - "I intend to understand the root cause of my anxiety and find ways to manage it better."

2. To enhance creativity:

  - "I aim to unlock my creative potential and generate new ideas for my art."

3. To experience a deeper connection with nature:

  - "I want to feel more connected to the natural world and appreciate its beauty."

4. To heal emotional wounds:

  - "I seek to confront and heal past traumas that have been holding me back."

5. To gain insight into a particular aspect of your life:

- "I hope to gain a deeper understanding of my career path and make informed decisions about my future."

Physical Preparation

Dietary Guidelines

What you eat before a psilocybin journey can significantly impact your experience. In the days leading up to your journey, consume clean and nutritious foods. Avoid alcohol and heavy, processed meals. On the day of your journey, eat light to prevent nausea. A light, healthy meal is recommended, avoiding heavy, greasy foods that can cause discomfort. Some people prefer fasting for a few hours before the journey to reduce nausea and enhance clarity.

Example of a Pre-Journey Meal Plan:

1. Two Days Before:

- Breakfast: Smoothie with spinach, banana, and almond milk
- Lunch: Quinoa salad with mixed vegetables and a light vinaigrette
- Dinner: Grilled salmon with steamed broccoli and brown rice

2. One Day Before:

- Breakfast: Oatmeal with fresh berries and honey
- Lunch: Turkey and avocado wrap with a side of carrot sticks
- Dinner: Baked chicken with sweet potatoes and green beans

3. Day of the Journey:

- Breakfast: Greek yogurt with a handful of nuts and seeds
- Light snacks if needed: Fresh fruit, raw nuts, or a small salad

Preparing Your Body

Preparing your body is essential for a positive psilocybin experience. Ensure you are well-rested, hydrated, and in good physical health. Engage in light exercise, stretch, and ensure you are well-rested. Physical well-being can positively influence your mental state and overall experience. Proper preparation can enhance the experience and help you handle the journey with more resilience and comfort.

Example of Pre-Journey Physical Preparation:

1. Exercise Routine:

- Morning yoga session focusing on deep stretches and relaxation
- A light jog or brisk walk in the afternoon to increase endorphins

2. Rest:

- Ensure you get at least 7-8 hours of sleep the night before your journey
- Take short naps if needed to feel fully rested

Hydration and Rest

Stay hydrated and get plenty of sleep the night before your journey. Being well-rested and hydrated helps ensure you are physically prepared for the experience.

Example of Hydration Plan:

1. Two Days Before:

- Drink at least 8 glasses of water throughout the day
- Avoid caffeinated and sugary drinks

2. One Day Before:

- Continue drinking at least 8 glasses of water

- Consider herbal teas like chamomile or peppermint for relaxation

3. Day of the Journey:

- Drink water regularly but avoid overhydration to prevent frequent bathroom trips

Mental and Emotional Preparation

Meditation and Mindfulness Practices

Regular meditation can help calm your mind and prepare you for the journey. Mindfulness practices can enhance your ability to stay present and navigate the experience with ease.

Example of a Meditation Routine:

1. Morning Meditation:

- Find a quiet place and sit comfortably
- Focus on your breath, inhaling deeply and exhaling slowly
- Spend 10-15 minutes clearing your mind and setting positive intentions

2. Evening Reflection:

- Reflect on your day and any emotions you experienced
- Practice gratitude by noting three things you are thankful for

Addressing Fears and Anxieties

Acknowledge any fears you may have and address them through journaling or talking with a trusted friend. Understanding and accepting your anxieties can help you feel more prepared and less apprehensive.

Example of Addressing Fears:

1. Journaling Exercise:

- Write down any fears or anxieties you have about the journey
- Reflect on the origins of these fears and how you can address them
- Create affirmations to counteract negative thoughts

2. Talking to a Friend:

- Share your concerns with a trusted friend who understands your intentions
- Discuss possible scenarios and how you might handle them
- Seek reassurance and support from your friend

Journaling Exercises

Write down your thoughts and feelings in the days leading up to the experience. Journaling can help you process emotions and clarify your intentions.

Example of Journaling Prompts:

1. Reflection on Intentions:

- What do I hope to gain from this experience?
- How can this journey help me achieve my goals?

2. Emotional Preparation:

- What emotions am I currently experiencing?
- How can I address any fears or anxieties I have about the journey?

3. Setting Goals:

- What specific outcomes do I desire from this journey?
- How will I know if I have achieved my intentions?

Setting the Environment

Creating a Safe Space

A safe and comfortable environment is vital for a psilocybin journey. Choose a quiet, comfortable, and familiar environment where you feel safe. Ensure that the space is free from distractions and interruptions, with comfortable seating or lying areas, calming lighting, and access to nature if possible. A safe space helps you feel secure, allowing you to fully immerse yourself in the experience.

Example of Creating a Safe Space:

1. Living Room Setup:

- Arrange comfortable seating with cushions and blankets
- Use soft, warm lighting like lamps or candles

- Ensure the room is clean and clutter-free

2. Outdoor Setup:

- Find a secluded spot in nature, like a garden or park
- Bring a comfortable chair or blanket to sit on
- Surround yourself with natural elements like plants, flowers, and water features

Choosing the Right Music

Prepare a playlist of soothing music to enhance your experience. Music can be a powerful tool in guiding and enriching your journey.

The Johns Hopkins playlist is a carefully curated selection of music designed to support and enhance the psilocybin experience. This playlist includes a range of genres and styles, chosen to guide and comfort you through different phases of your journey. Many find it helpful to use this playlist as a backdrop to their experience.

Example of a Psilocybin Journey Playlist:

1. Ambient Music:

- "Weightless" by Marconi Union
- "A Moment of Stillness" by God Is An Astronaut

2. Nature Sounds:

- "Forest Sounds" by Nature Soundscapes
- "Ocean Waves" by Relaxing White Noise

3. Instrumental Tracks:

- "Clair de Lune" by Debussy
- "Spiegel im Spiegel" by Arvo Pärt

Essential Items to Have

- Comfortable clothing
- Blankets and pillows
- Water and light snacks
- A journal and pen
- Meaningful objects (e.g., crystals, photos)

Example of Essential Items:

1. Comfortable Clothing:

- Loose-fitting, soft fabrics like cotton or linen
- Layers to adjust to temperature changes

2. Snacks:

- Fresh fruit like apples or berries
- Nuts and seeds for protein
- Herbal teas for hydration

Having essential items like water, snacks, a journal, and a blanket can significantly enhance your comfort and safety during the journey. Water and snacks help maintain hydration and energy levels, while a journal allows you to document insights and experiences. A blanket can provide warmth and comfort, contributing to a sense of security.

Part Two: The Journey

Dosing

Determining the Right Dose

For beginners, it's crucial to start with a low to moderate dose. A typical starting dose is between 1 to 1.5 grams of dried mushrooms. This dosage range allows you to gauge your sensitivity and reaction to psilocybin in a controlled manner. Experienced individuals may opt for higher doses, but this guide focuses on beginners to ensure a safe and positive experience.

Factors Affecting Dosage

- Body Weight: Heavier individuals may require slightly higher doses to achieve the same effects.
- Sensitivity: Everyone's body reacts differently to psilocybin. Start low and adjust as necessary for future experiences.
- Set and Setting: Your mental state and environment can influence the intensity of the experience. Ensure both are positive and supportive.

Microdosing

What is Microdosing

Microdosing involves taking sub-perceptual doses of psilocybin, typically around 0.1 to 0.3 grams of dried mushrooms. This practice aims to provide the benefits of psilocybin, such as enhanced mood and creativity, without inducing a full psychedelic experience.

Benefits of Microdosing

- Improved mood and emotional stability
- Enhanced focus and productivity
- Increased creativity and problem-solving skills
- Reduced symptoms of depression and anxiety

Microdosing Schedule

A common schedule is to take a microdose every three days, allowing your body to integrate the benefits without building tolerance. Adjust the schedule based on your personal experience and needs.

Example of a Microdosing Schedule:

1. Day 1:

   - Take 0.1 grams of dried mushrooms with breakfast

- Monitor your mood and productivity throughout the day

2. Day 2:

   - No microdose
   - Reflect on the previous day's experience in your journal

3. Day 3:

   - No microdose
   - Continue to monitor your mood and productivity

4. Day 4:

   - Repeat the microdose and journaling process

Consumption Methods

Different Methods of Consumption

Psilocybin can be consumed in various forms, each with its unique advantages. Choose the method that feels most comfortable and natural for you.

Dried Mushrooms

The most common method is to consume dried mushrooms directly. They can be eaten as they are, but some people find the taste unpleasant.

- Pros: Easy and straightforward.
- Cons: Taste can be unpleasant; may cause nausea.

Different individuals have unique ways of consuming psilocybin mushrooms to enhance their experience and manage any discomfort.

For example:

Some people prefer to chew dried mushrooms slowly and follow up with a sip of water to wash down the taste. They find it helpful to eat a small piece of ginger to combat any nausea.

Capsules

Capsules containing psilocybin powder are another popular method. They allow for precise dosing and eliminate the taste issue.

- Pros: Precise dosing, no taste.
- Cons: Requires preparation or purchase from a reliable source.

Psilocybin Tea

Making tea from psilocybin mushrooms is a gentler method on the stomach and can be flavored to improve taste.

- Pros: Easier on the stomach, can mask taste.
- Cons: Requires preparation.

Example:

Some people prefer to grind their dried mushrooms into a fine powder and steep them in hot water with a slice of lemon and honey. They find the tea soothing and enjoy the ritual of preparation.

Edibles

Psilocybin mushrooms can be incorporated into various edibles, such as chocolates or baked goods.

- Pros: Can mask the taste completely, enjoyable experience.
- Cons: Requires preparation, may alter potency.

Example:

Some people make psilocybin-infused chocolate truffles. they follow a recipe that ensures even distribution of the psilocybin and enjoy this sweet treat as part of thier journey.

Preparing Psilocybin Tea

1. Grind the Mushrooms: Use a grinder to break down the dried mushrooms into a fine powder.

2. Boil Water: Bring water to a boil and then let it cool slightly.

3. Steep the Mushrooms: Pour the hot water over the mushroom powder and let it steep for 10-15 minutes.

4. Strain and Serve: Strain the mixture to remove any solid particles, and enjoy your tea.

Example:

Others prefer to add ginger and chamomile to their psilocybin tea to enhance the flavor and reduce any potential nausea.

What to Expect

Feelings and Visuals at Different Dose Ranges

The effects of psilocybin can vary significantly based on the dosage. Here is a general guide to what you might expect at different dose ranges:

1. Microdose (0.1 to 0.3 grams)
   - Feelings: Slight uplift in mood, increased focus, enhanced creativity, and mild euphoria.
   - Visuals: Generally, no visual hallucinations. You may notice slight enhancements in color perception and visual acuity.

Example:

Emily takes a microdose before her workday. She feels a subtle increase in her energy levels and finds herself more focused and creative during her tasks.

2. Low Dose (0.5 to 1 gram)

- Feelings: Mild euphoria, heightened senses, increased empathy, and introspective thoughts.
- Visuals: Colors may appear brighter, and patterns may seem more vivid. No significant hallucinations.

Example:

Alex takes 0.7 grams of dried mushrooms and spends the afternoon in a park. He feels more connected to nature and notices the vibrant colors of the flowers and trees.

3. Moderate Dose (1 to 2 grams)

- Feelings: Stronger euphoria, emotional release, deeper introspection, and a sense of interconnectedness.
- Visuals: Light to moderate visual hallucinations, including geometric patterns, enhanced colors, and slight distortions in perception.

Example:

Maria takes 1.5 grams of dried mushrooms and listens to her favorite music. She experiences emotional release and gains new insights into her personal relationships.

4. High Dose (2 to 3.5 grams)

- Feelings: Intense euphoria, profound emotional experiences, significant introspection, and possible spiritual insights.
- Visuals: Strong visual hallucinations, including complex geometric patterns, vibrant colors, and changes in perception of time and space.

Example: Jason takes 3 grams of dried mushrooms and has a deeply spiritual experience. He feels a profound sense of unity with the universe and gains insights into his life's purpose.

5. Heroic Dose (4 grams and above)

- Feelings: Extremely intense emotional and spiritual experiences, possible ego dissolution, and a sense of transcendence.
- Visuals: Extremely vivid and immersive visual hallucinations, including seeing entities, out-of-

body experiences, and a complete alteration of reality.

Example:

Samantha takes 5 grams of dried mushrooms in a controlled, safe setting. She experiences ego dissolution and gains profound spiritual insights that change her perspective on life.

During the Experience

What to Expect During Different Stages of the Journey

1. Onset (20-60 minutes)

- Feelings: Initial sensations may include a sense of anticipation, slight nervousness, or excitement. Physical sensations like tingling or a light body buzz may occur.
- Visuals: Subtle changes in perception, such as enhanced colors and patterns.

Example:

During the onset, You may feel a slight tingling in his hands and a growing sense of excitement. He notices the colors in his room becoming more vibrant.

2. Peak (2-4 hours)

- Feelings: The peak is the most intense part of the journey, characterized by strong emotional and sensory experiences. Euphoria, deep introspection, and a sense of interconnectedness are common.
- Visuals: Vivid visual hallucinations, including geometric patterns, shifting shapes, and enhanced colors. Objects may appear to breathe or move.

Example:

At the peak of your journey, You may feel waves of euphoria and a profound sense of connection to the universe. You may see intricate patterns and colors swirling around you.

3. Plateau (2-4 hours)

- Feelings: The intensity of the peak subsides, leading to a more stable but still significant level of experience. Emotional and sensory experiences remain heightened but less overwhelming.

- Visuals: Visuals continue but are less intense than
  during the peak. Patterns and colors remain
  vibrant, but movement and distortions decrease.

Example:

During the plateau, You may feel a sense of calm and
contentment. The visual patterns are still present but less
intense, allowing you to reflect on your insights.

4. Come Down (1-2 hours)

- Feelings: A gradual return to normal
  consciousness, with lingering feelings of peace,
  introspection, and mild euphoria. Some
  individuals may feel tired or introspective.
- Visuals: Visuals fade, and perception returns to
  normal. Mild aftereffects, such as enhanced
  appreciation of colors, may persist.

Example:

As the journey comes to an end, You may feel a sense
of peace and relaxation. The visuals fade, and you can
reflect on your experience with gratitude.

Techniques for Staying Grounded

Focus on your breath, listen to music, or hold a comforting object to stay grounded. Remind yourself that the experience is temporary and will eventually pass.

Example of Grounding Techniques:

1. Breathing Exercise:

- Sit comfortably and close your eyes
- Inhale deeply for a count of four, hold for a count of four, exhale for a count of four
- Repeat this cycle for several minutes until you feel calm

2. Music:

- Listen to calming instrumental music or nature sounds
- Focus on the rhythm and melody to anchor your thoughts

3. Comfort Objects:

- Hold a soft blanket or a favorite stuffed animal
- Focus on the texture and sensation to bring yourself back to the present moment

Handling Challenging Moments

If you encounter difficult moments, remind yourself that the experience is temporary and focus on your breath. It can also help to change your environment slightly, such as moving to another room or adjusting the lighting.

Example of Handling Challenging Moments:

1. Change Your Environment:

- Move to a different room with softer lighting
- Open a window to let in fresh air and natural sounds

2. Positive Affirmations:

- Repeat calming phrases like, "I am safe," "This will pass," or "I am in control."
- Write these affirmations down and keep them nearby as reminders

3. Guided Meditation:

- Listen to a guided meditation track designed for psilocybin journeys
- Follow the voice and visualize calming scenes to shift your focus

Role of a Sitter

Importance of a Sitter

A sitter can provide reassurance and help you stay safe during the journey. They serve as a grounded presence, offering support if needed.

Choosing the Right Sitter

Select someone you trust, who is calm and experienced with psychedelics. Ensure they understand their role and responsibilities.

Example of a Sitter's Role:

1. Supportive Presence:

- Sit quietly in the same room or nearby, ready to assist if needed
- Offer comforting words and physical touch if appropriate

2. Monitoring:

- Keep an eye on the individual's physical and emotional state

- Be prepared to intervene if they become distressed or disoriented

3. Guidance:

- Help the individual stay grounded with breathing exercises or conversation
- Provide reassurance and remind them of their intentions and safety

Responsibilities of a Sitter

The sitter should remain sober and be available to assist you throughout the experience. They should provide comfort, reassurance, and help you navigate any challenging moments.

Example of a Sitter's Actions:

1. Before the Journey:

- Discuss the individual's intentions and any specific concerns
- Plan out the session, including setting up the environment and preparing necessary items

2. During the Journey:

- Stay attentive and responsive to the individual's needs

- Offer gentle guidance and reassurance without being intrusive

3. After the Journey:

- Help the individual reflect on their experience and journal their insights
- Provide ongoing support and encourage healthy integration practices

Part Three: Integration

Immediate Post-Experience

Reflecting on the Journey

Take time to reflect on your experience through journaling or talking with a friend. Reflecting helps consolidate the insights gained during the journey.

Example of Reflection:

1. Journaling Prompts:

- What were the most significant moments of my journey?
- How did I feel during the peak of the experience?
- What insights or realizations did I have?

2. Talking with a Friend:

- Share key highlights and emotions from the journey
- Discuss any challenges faced and how they were managed
- Seek feedback and support from your friend

Self-Care Practices

Engage in gentle activities like yoga, walking, or taking a bath. Self-care practices can help you feel grounded and nurtured after the experience.

Example of Self-Care Practices:

1. Gentle Yoga:

- Practice restorative poses like child's pose, legs up the wall, and savasana
- Focus on deep breathing and relaxation

2. Nature Walk:

- Take a walk in a nearby park or natural area
- Pay attention to the sights, sounds, and smells around you to stay present

3. Warm Bath:

- Add Epsom salts or essential oils to the bath for added relaxation
- Soak for 20-30 minutes while listening to calming music

Grounding Techniques

Practice grounding exercises such as deep breathing or connecting with nature. These techniques can help you feel centered and balanced.Example of Grounding Techniques:

1. Deep Breathing:

- Sit or lie down comfortably
- Inhale deeply through your nose, hold for a few seconds, then exhale slowly through your mouth
- Repeat this process several times until you feel grounded

2. Connecting with Nature:

- Walk barefoot on grass or sand to feel the earth beneath your feet
- Spend time gardening or tending to plants
- Sit quietly in a natural setting and observe your surroundings
-

Long-Term Integration

Incorporating Insights into Daily Life

Identify ways to apply the insights gained from your journey to your everyday life. Integration is about making meaningful changes and incorporating new perspectives.

Example of Incorporating Insights:

1. Personal Growth:

- Set new goals based on the realizations from your journey

- Develop a daily mindfulness or meditation practice

2. Relationships:

- Communicate more openly and honestly with loved ones
- Practice active listening and empathy in your interactions

3. Lifestyle Changes:

- Adopt healthier habits, such as regular exercise, balanced nutrition, and adequate sleep
- Explore new hobbies or creative outlets that align with your passions

Continued Mindfulness and Meditation

Maintain a regular meditation practice to keep the benefits of the experience alive. Mindfulness can help you stay connected to the insights and growth achieved during your journey.

Example of a Meditation Routine:

1. Daily Practice:

- Set aside 10-20 minutes each morning for meditation

- Focus on your breath and observe your thoughts
  without judgment

2. Mindfulness Exercises:

- Practice mindful eating by savoring each bite and
  paying attention to the flavors and textures
- Engage in mindful walking by focusing on the
  sensations of each step and your surroundings

Seeking Support if Needed

Consider joining a support group or seeking professional
help if you struggle with integration. There are many
resources available to support your ongoing journey.

Example of Seeking Support:

1. Support Groups:

- Join online forums or local groups focused on
  psychedelic integration
- Attend meetings and share your experiences with
  others who understand

2. Professional Help:

- Seek a therapist or counselor experienced in
  psychedelic integration
- Participate in integration workshops or retreats

Sharing Your Experience

Talking with Friends and Family

Share your experience with trusted individuals who can offer support. Talking about your journey can help you process and integrate the experience.

Example of Sharing Your Experience:

1. Close Friends:

- Choose friends who are open-minded and supportive
- Share key insights and emotions from your journey
- Be honest about any challenges faced and how you overcame them

2. Family Members:

- Approach family members who may be interested or supportive
- Explain your intentions and the positive outcomes of your journey
- Be patient and open to their questions and concerns

Joining Support Groups

Connect with others who have had similar experiences. Support groups can provide a sense of community and understanding.

Example of Joining Support Groups:

1. Online Communities:

- Join forums like Reddit's r/Psychedelics or The Third Wave's community
- Participate in discussions, ask questions, and share your experiences

2. Local Groups:

- Look for local meetup groups or organizations focused on psychedelic integration
- Attend meetings, workshops, and events to connect with others

Creative Expression

Express your journey through art, writing, or other creative outlets. Creativity can be a powerful way to process and share your insights.

Example of Creative Expression:

1. Art:

- Create paintings, drawings, or sculptures that reflect your experience
- Use colors, shapes, and symbols to convey your emotions and insights

2. Writing:

- Write poems, stories, or essays about your journey
- Start a blog or journal to document your ongoing integration process

3. Music:

- Compose songs or create playlists that capture the essence of your experience
- Share your music with friends or online communities

Part Four: Managing Difficult Experiences

Understanding Bad Trips

What is a Bad Trip?

A bad trip refers to a challenging or negative experience while under the influence of psilocybin. This can include feelings of fear, anxiety, paranoia, or overwhelming emotions. It's important to understand that bad trips can happen, and knowing how to handle them can make a significant difference.

Common Triggers for Bad Trips

- Set and Setting: An uncomfortable environment or negative mindset can contribute to a bad trip.
- High Dosage: Taking too high a dose, especially for beginners, can lead to an overwhelming experience.
- Emotional State: Existing anxiety, stress, or unresolved emotional issues can be amplified during a trip.

Example of a Bad Trip:

Laura, a 28-year-old graphic designer, took a high dose of psilocybin without proper preparation. She found herself overwhelmed by intense emotions and vivid hallucinations, leading to feelings of fear and panic. By understanding what triggered her bad trip, she was able to approach future journeys with better preparation and lower doses.

Preventing Bad Trips

Preparation

Thorough preparation is key to preventing bad trips. Follow the guidelines in this guide for setting intentions, preparing your body and mind, and creating a safe environment.

Example of Preparation:

1. Set Clear Intentions:

- Write down your goals and hopes for the journey
- Reflect on these intentions regularly leading up to the experience

2. Prepare Your Environment:

- Ensure your space is comfortable, safe, and free from distractions
- Gather essential items like blankets, water, and comforting objects

3. Mind and Body Preparation:

- Engage in meditation, journaling, and light exercise
- Eat clean, nutritious foods and stay hydrated

Start with a Low Dose

Begin with a low dose to gauge your sensitivity and reaction to psilocybin. Gradually increase the dose in future experiences if desired.

Example of Starting with a Low Dose:

1. First-Time User:

- Take 1 gram of dried mushrooms
- Monitor your response and adjust accordingly in future journeys

2. Gradual Increase:

- If comfortable, increase to 1.5 grams on a subsequent journey
- Continue to adjust based on your experiences and comfort level

Choose the Right Environment

Ensure you are in a comfortable, familiar, and safe space. Avoid environments with potential distractions or stressors.

Example of Creating a Safe Environment:

1. Indoor Space:

- Set up a cozy room with soft lighting,
  comfortable seating, and calming music
- Ensure the space is clean, clutter-free, and free
  from interruptions

2. Outdoor Space:

- Choose a secluded spot in nature with minimal
  disturbances
- Bring a blanket or chair, and surround yourself
  with natural beauty

Have a Trusted Sitter

Having a sober, experienced sitter can provide
reassurance and help you navigate any challenging
moments.

Example of a Sitter's Role:

1. Before the Journey:

- Discuss the individual's intentions and any
  specific concerns
- Plan out the session, including setting up the
  environment and preparing necessary items

2. During the Journey:

- Stay attentive and responsive to the individual's
  needs
- Offer gentle guidance and reassurance without
  being intrusive

3. After the Journey:

- Help the individual reflect on their experience
  and journal their insights
- Provide ongoing support and encourage healthy
  integration practices
-

Handling Bad Trips

Stay Calm and Breathe

If you find yourself experiencing a bad trip, focus on
your breath. Deep, slow breathing can help calm your
mind and body.

Example of Staying Calm:

1. Breathing Exercise:

- Sit comfortably and close your eyes
- Inhale deeply for a count of four, hold for a count
  of four, exhale for a count of four
- Repeat this cycle for several minutes until you
  feel calm

2. Positive Affirmations:

- Repeat calming phrases like, "I am safe," "This
  will pass," or "I am in control."
- Write these affirmations down and keep them
  nearby as reminders

Change Your Environment

If possible, move to a different room or adjust the lighting. Sometimes a change in environment can shift your perspective and reduce anxiety.

Example of Changing Your Environment:

1. Move to a Different Room:

- Find a room with softer lighting or natural light
- Open a window to let in fresh air and natural sounds

2. Adjust Lighting:

- Dim the lights or use a soft lamp to create a calming atmosphere
- Avoid harsh or bright lights that can exacerbate anxiety

Talk to Your Sitter

Communicate with your sitter about what you're experiencing. They can offer comfort, reassurance, and help you feel grounded.

Example of Talking to Your Sitter:

1. Share Your Feelings:

- Explain what you're experiencing and any specific fears or anxieties
- Allow your sitter to offer reassurance and support

2. Seek Guidance:

- Ask your sitter for grounding exercises or calming activities
- Follow their guidance to help navigate challenging moments

Remind Yourself It's Temporary

Remember that the experience is temporary and will eventually pass. Reassuring yourself of this can help you stay calm.

Example of Reminding Yourself:

1. Positive Self-Talk:

- Repeat phrases like, "This is temporary," "I will get through this," or "I am safe."
- Focus on the temporary nature of the experience and the positive outcomes

2. Visualize the End:

- Imagine yourself coming out of the experience feeling refreshed and insightful

- Visualize the positive outcomes and how you will integrate them into your life

Engage in Soothing Activities

Listen to calming music, hold a comforting object, or engage in gentle activities like drawing or coloring.

Example of Soothing Activities:

1. Calming Music:

- Listen to ambient or instrumental music with a slow tempo
- Focus on the rhythm and melody to anchor your thoughts

2. Comfort Objects:

- Hold a soft blanket, a favorite stuffed animal, or a comforting piece of jewelry
- Focus on the texture and sensation to bring yourself back to the present moment

3. Gentle Activities:

- Draw or color in a coloring book to engage your mind and hands
- Write in a journal or sketch your feelings and experiences

Counteracting a Psilocybin Trip

Is it Possible to Stop a Trip?

Unlike substances like alcohol or opioids, there is no direct antidote to counteract a psilocybin trip. However, there are ways to manage and reduce the intensity of the experience.

Hydration and Nutrition

Drinking water and eating light snacks can help stabilize your body and mind. Avoid caffeine or other stimulants.

Example of Hydration and Nutrition:

1. Drink Water:

- Sip water regularly to stay hydrated
- Avoid caffeinated or sugary drinks

2. Light Snacks:

- Eat fresh fruit, raw nuts, or a small salad
- Avoid heavy or processed foods

Grounding Techniques

Engage in grounding exercises, such as touching a familiar object, walking barefoot on grass, or focusing on your breath.

Example of Grounding Techniques:

1. Touch Familiar Objects:

- Hold a favorite blanket, stuffed animal, or piece of jewelry
- Focus on the texture and sensation to bring yourself back to the present moment

2. Walk Barefoot:

- Walk on grass, sand, or other natural surfaces to feel the earth beneath your feet
- Pay attention to the sensations and connect with nature

Pharmacological Interventions

In extreme cases, a medical professional may administer medications such as benzodiazepines to reduce anxiety and calm the individual. This should only be done under medical supervision.

Example of Pharmacological Interventions:

1. Seek Medical Help:

- If the situation becomes unmanageable or if there are signs of physical distress, seek medical assistance immediately
- A healthcare professional can provide appropriate interventions and support

Seeking Medical Help

If the situation becomes unmanageable or if there are any signs of physical distress, seek medical assistance immediately.

Example of Seeking Medical Help:

1. Emergency Response:

- Call emergency services if you or someone else is in distress
- Provide clear information about the situation and any substances involved

2. Follow Medical Advice:

- Follow the guidance of medical professionals to ensure safety and well-being
- Be honest about the substances used and any symptoms experienced

Conclusion

Embarking on a psilocybin journey is a profound and transformative experience that can offer deep insights, healing, and personal growth. As you step into this journey, remember that preparation is key. By setting clear intentions, preparing your body, considering your diet, and creating a safe and comfortable environment, you lay the foundation for a meaningful and enriching experience.

Music, such as the Johns Hopkins playlist, can enhance your journey, guiding you through the various phases of the experience. Having essential items like water, snacks, a journal, and a blanket will ensure your comfort and safety throughout the journey.

During the experience, staying present and open to whatever arises is crucial. Each journey is unique, and by approaching it with respect and mindfulness, you can unlock its full potential.

As you integrate the insights and lessons from your psilocybin journey into your daily life, give yourself time to reflect and process. Journaling, talking with trusted friends, or seeking professional guidance can help you make sense of your experiences and apply the newfound wisdom to your personal growth and well-being.

Remember, the journey doesn't end with the psilocybin experience itself. It's an ongoing process of learning, healing, and evolving. Embrace the changes, trust in your path, and continue to cultivate the awareness and insights gained during your journey.

Thank you for choosing this guide to accompany you on your psilocybin journey. May it serve as a valuable resource, offering support, knowledge, and inspiration as you explore the profound depths of your consciousness.

Safe travels, and may your journey be filled with wonder, insight, and transformation.

Resources

Fireside Project

The Fireside Project is a nonprofit organization dedicated to providing peer support during psychedelic experiences. Their services are designed to help individuals navigate challenging moments, integrate insights, and ensure a safe and positive journey. Below is some essential information about the Fireside Project and how you can reach out to them for support.

About Fireside Project:

The Fireside Project offers a free, confidential, and compassionate support line for individuals undergoing psychedelic experiences. Trained volunteers are available to provide emotional support, guidance, and information to help you through your journey. Whether you are preparing for a psychedelic experience, currently navigating one, or integrating the insights afterward, the Fireside Project is here to help.

Services Provided:

- o Peer support during psychedelic experiences
- o Guidance and reassurance during challenging moments

o   Integration support to help process and
    understand your experience
o   Confidential and non-judgmental listening

How to Reach Fireside Project:

o   **Support Line Number:** 62-FIRESIDE (623-473-7433)
o   **Website:** firesideproject.org
o   **Availability:** The support line operates daily, providing timely assistance to those in need.
o   **Contact Methods:** You can call or text the support line at 62-FIRESIDE (623-473-7433).

Why Use Fireside Project:

o   **Confidential and Compassionate:** Your conversations are private, and the volunteers are trained to provide empathetic and non-judgmental support.
o   **Experienced Volunteers:** The support team consists of individuals with experience in navigating psychedelic experiences, offering practical advice and emotional comfort.
o   **Accessible and Free:** The service is free of charge, making it accessible to everyone who needs support during their psychedelic journey.

How to Prepare:

Before reaching out to the Fireside Project, it's helpful to:

- o Be in a quiet and safe environment where you can talk openly.
- o Have basic information about your psychedelic experience ready, such as the substance, dosage, and time of ingestion.
- o Be open and honest about what you are experiencing and how you are feeling.

The Fireside Project is committed to supporting you through every stage of your psychedelic journey, ensuring that you feel heard, understood, and cared for. Whether you need immediate assistance or ongoing support for integration, their dedicated team is ready to help.

For more information, visit firesideproject.org or call or text their support line at 62-FIRESIDE (623-473-7433).

Quick Reference Sheet

Psilocybin Dosage Guide

- **Microdose**: 0.1 - 0.3 grams
- **Low Dose**: 0.5 - 1 gram
- **Moderate Dose**: 1 - 1.5 grams
- **Standard Dose:** 2 - 3.5 grams
- **High Dose:** 4 - 5 grams

Quick Tips

- **Duration of Effects:**
  - **Micro to Standard Doses:** 4-6 hours
  - **High Dose:** 6-8 hours
- **Onset Time:** 20-60 minutes
- **Peak Effects:** 2-3 hours after ingestion
- **Set and Setting:** Calm, comfortable, familiar environment
- **Essential Items:** Water, snacks, journal, blanket
- **Integration:** Reflect, journal, discuss your experience
- **Hydration:** Drink water before and after the journey

- **Safety:** Have a trusted friend or sitter present if possible

Positive Mindset

- **Affirmations**: Use positive affirmations to set your mindset
- **Breathing**: Practice deep breathing to stay calm
- **Acceptance**:Embrace whatever arises during the journey

Sensory Enhancements

- **Music**: Use calming music like the Johns Hopkins playlist
- **Lighting**: Soft, ambient lighting enhances comfort
- **Nature**:Access to nature can be grounding and soothing